THE VEGETARIAN BARIATRIC DIET COOKBOOK

Gastric Sleeve Plant Based Recipes to Stay slim, Overcome Food Addiction and Maintain Healthy Lifestyle Before and After Weight-Loss Surgery

Cynthia R. Perry

TABLE OF CONTENTS

INTRODUCTION

My stepmother was a middle-aged woman with a soft voice and a kind face. She had always been a bit overweight, but recently her weight had ballooned and she was struggling to keep up with her daily activities. She was embarrassed and ashamed of her appearance, and she had even stopped going to church because she felt so uncomfortable in her own skin.

One day, she was scrolling through her social media feeds when an article for a bariatric diet caught her eye. She had heard of diets like these before, but she had never considered actually trying one. However, something about the article made her stop and take notice. She decided that she would give it a try and see if it could help her.

The next day, she went to the store and picked up the supplies for the vegetarian bariatric diet. She had been a vegetarian for years, so she was already familiar with many of the foods she would be eating. She knew that she would need to be very disciplined in order to make the diet work, but she was determined to make it happen.

For the first week of the diet, She stuck to the guidelines and ate only the foods that were recommended. She was careful to measure out her portions and to drink plenty of water. She also tried to get in some exercise each day, even if it was just a walk around the block.

After the first week, my stepmother started to feel a difference in her body. She had more energy and felt less bloated. She was also starting to look more toned and fit. She was excited at the prospect of continuing the diet and seeing even more progress.

Each week, she followed the plan and continued to make progress. After a few months, she had lost a significant amount of weight and was feeling more confident in her own skin. She had also started to take up new activities like yoga and swimming, which she had avoided before due to her weight.

Her experience with the vegetarian bariatric diet was a true success story. She was able to reverse her situation and improve her health and self-esteem. She was proud of herself for having the courage and determination to stick with the diet, even when it was difficult.

She was so inspired by her success that she started to share her story with others. She was able to encourage other people to give the diet a try, and she was happy to be able to help them in their own weight loss journeys. She had found a way to turn her life around and she was determined to help others do the same.

My stepmother's success story is a testament to the power of the vegetarian bariatric diet. With dedication and determination, she was able to take back control of her body and her life. She is now healthier, happier, and more confident than ever before.

Chapter 1

Basics of Bariatric Surgery

Bariatric surgery is a type of weight loss procedure designed to help individuals who are severely obese lose weight and improve their health. It works by restricting the amount of food the stomach can hold, resulting in a decrease in calorie intake and aiding in weight loss. The procedure can also reduce the absorption of nutrients from food, as well as hormones that regulate hunger and satiety.

Bariatric surgery is typically recommended for individuals who are at least 100 pounds overweight or have a body mass index (BMI) of 40 or higher. It is also recommended for those with a BMI of 35 or higher, who also suffer from a related medical condition, such as diabetes, high blood pressure, or sleep apnea.

It works by reducing the size of the stomach and/or bypassing part of the small intestine. This limits the amount of food you can eat and reduces the number of calories and nutrients your body absorbs. This leads to gradual, sustained weight loss.

Bariatric surgery is typically done laparoscopically, using small incisions and a camera to view the stomach and other organs. The surgeon will remove a portion of the stomach, creating a smaller pouch. This pouch is then connected directly to the small intestine, bypassing most of the stomach. This reduces the size of the stomach, which limits the amount of food the patient can consume.

Common Types of Bariatric Surgery

The two most common types of bariatric surgery are Roux-en-Y Gastric Bypass and Sleeve Gastrectomy.

- **Roux-en-Y Gastric Bypass**

Roux-en-Y gastric bypass, also known as gastric bypass, is a type of bariatric surgery used to treat morbid obesity. The procedure creates a small stomach pouch that is connected to the small intestine, bypassing the larger stomach and upper portion of the small intestine. This limits the amount of food the patient can eat, as well as reduces their calorie absorption.

The Roux-en-Y gastric bypass procedure is one of the most commonly performed bariatric surgeries. It has been used successfully to help patients achieve significant weight loss and improve their health. Patients typically experience a decrease in hunger, as well as an improvement in nutrition, due to the bypass. Additionally, Roux-en-Y gastric bypass can reduce the risk of ccrtain medical conditions, such as type 2 diabetes and sleep apnea.

Although Roux-en-Y gastric bypass is an effective and safe weight-loss surgery, it is major surgery and carries associated risks. Patients should be aware that it is an irreversible procedure, and that there may be long-term side effects. These can include vitamin and mineral deficiencies, stomach pain, nausea, hair loss, and low blood sugar. It is important to discuss any possible risks with a doctor before deciding on surgery.

It is also important to recognize that even after surgery, patients must still adhere to a healthy diet and exercise regimen to maintain their weight loss. As with any weight-loss procedure, the results of Roux-en-Y gastric bypass vary from person to person, and it is important to work with a doctor to ensure the best possible outcome.

- **Sleeve Gastrectomy**

Sleeve gastrectomy is a type of bariatric surgery used to treat obesity. It is a more permanent, restrictive form of weight loss surgery compared to adjustable gastric banding, and involves removing a large portion of the stomach permanently.

Sleeve gastrectomy is done laparoscopically, which means the surgeon operates without making any large incisions. During the procedure, the surgeon removes about 75 percent of the stomach and creates a new, tube-shaped stomach, or "sleeve." This smaller stomach can hold less food, so people feel full faster and eat less.

The main benefit of sleeve gastrectomy is that it helps people lose weight and improve their overall health. People who have had the procedure often report a dramatic decrease in appetite and a significant reduction in the amount of food they can eat. This leads to significant and sustained weight loss.

In addition to weight loss, sleeve gastrectomy can also reduce the risk of developing conditions such as diabetes, heart disease, and high blood pressure. It can also improve quality of life by reducing the impact of obesity-related physical and psychological issues.

Sleeve gastrectomy is a safe procedure, but it does come with some risks. Complications can include infection, leakage, and bleeding. Additionally, the procedure is not reversible, so it is important to consider the long-term consequences before committing to the surgery.

Overall, sleeve gastrectomy is a safe and effective way to treat obesity. It can help people lose weight, reduce their risk of developing certain conditions, and improve their quality of life. However, it is important to talk to a doctor to determine if this type of surgery is the right choice for you.

Bariatric surgery is a major step in the process of weight loss and requires a commitment to lifestyle changes.

This surgery is generally safe and effective, but it is important to understand the risks associated with the procedure. Complications can include infection, blood clots, and a leak in the stomach or intestine. Patients may also experience nausea, vomiting, and diarrhea. It is important to discuss the risks and benefits of the procedure with a qualified physician before deciding to undergo bariatric surgery.

In addition to the potential risks, it is also important to understand the lifestyle changes that must be made to ensure successful weight loss after bariatric surgery. Patients must follow a strict diet plan, including eating smaller, frequent meals and avoiding certain foods. You must also exercise regularly and make healthy lifestyle changes, such as quitting smoking and reducing alcohol consumption.

These changes are necessary for the success and long-term maintenance of the weight loss achieved with bariatric surgery.

Chapter 2

Understanding Vegetarian Bariatric Cooking

Vegetarian Bariatric cooking is a type of cooking that focuses on the dietary needs of individuals who have had bariatric surgery. This type of cooking provides meals that are low in calories, fat, and carbohydrates, while still being nutrient-dense and flavorful. The goal of vegetarian bariatric cooking is to create meals that are healthy and satisfying for individuals who have had bariatric surgery, without sacrificing taste.

Vegetarian Bariatric cooking is based on the principles of a healthy, balanced diet. The emphasis is on plant-based foods, such as vegetables, fruits, grains, nuts, and legumes. This type of cooking also includes lean proteins, such as beans, tofu, and tempeh, to provide a complete protein source. Fats are limited to healthy sources, such as olive oil, avocados, and nuts.

Meals should include a variety of nutrient-dense foods to provide the body with all the necessary vitamins and minerals. Vegetables should be the focus of any meal, as they are low in calories and packed with vitamins, minerals, and fiber. Fruits, nuts, and legumes should be included for their high nutrient content and for their ability to help keep you feeling full. Whole grains and lean proteins should also be included to provide the body with energy and protein to help keep you feeling full for longer.

When cooking for a vegetarian Bariatric diet, it is important to choose foods that are low in sodium, fat, and added sugars. Eating low-sodium, low-fat, and low-sugar foods can help to reduce the risk of developing health problems such as high blood pressure, heart disease, and diabetes. A low-sodium, low-fat, and low-sugar diet can help people who have had bariatric surgery lose weight and maintain their weight loss.

Eating these types of foods can help to reduce hunger and cravings, which can make it easier to stick to a healthy eating plan. Eating low-sodium, low-fat, and low-sugar foods can also help to reduce inflammation in the body, which can help to improve overall health and well-being.

For vegetarian bariatric cooking, it is important to focus on eating fresh and unprocessed foods to get the most nutrition. This includes choosing lean proteins, whole grains, and plenty of fruits and vegetables. It is also important to limit processed and packaged foods that are high in sodium, fat and added sugars.

Processed and packaged foods should be avoided, as these can be high in sodium and added sugars. Instead, fresh and frozen fruits and vegetables, as well as whole grains, nuts, and legumes, should be used.

It is also important to pay attention to portion sizes when cooking for a vegetarian Bariatric diet. Portion control is an essential aspect of any weight-loss diet, and vegetarian bariatric diets are no exception. Eating smaller portions allows for weight loss without feeling deprived. Smaller portions also help to make sure that your vegetarian bariatric diet is balanced and nutrient dense.

For vegetarians, portion size can be especially important because the diet typically lacks certain nutrients that are found in meat and fish. Therefore, larger portions of vegetarian foods may not provide sufficient amounts of essential nutrients. With a vegetarian bariatric diet, portion size helps to ensure that the individual is receiving enough of the nutrients they need while still maintaining a calorie deficit.

Additionally, portion size can help to reduce overeating and establish healthy eating habits. Consuming smaller portions can prevent overeating and help to create a sense of satisfaction when eating. This can help individuals to become more mindful of their food choices and reduce the temptation to overeat

The portions should be small and the meals should be spread out throughout the day. Eating several small meals throughout the day can help to keep hunger at bay and can help to ensure that the body is getting all the necessary nutrients.

Cooking for a vegetarian Bariatric diet doesn't have to be complicated or time-consuming. With a bit of planning and creativity, meals can be tasty and nutritious. Some ideas for quick and easy vegetarian Bariatric meals include vegetable stir-fries, lentil soups, quinoa salads, and roasted vegetables. There are also plenty of delicious vegetarian recipes that can be easily adapted to fit a Bariatric diet.

The Benefits of a Vegetarian Diet

Vegetarian diets are becoming increasingly popular as a lifestyle choice, and for those looking to manage their weight, they can be especially beneficial. Bariatric cooking, or cooking for those who have undergone weight loss surgery, often relies heavily on a vegetarian diet due to its lower calorie content and higher nutrient density.

One of the main benefits of a vegetarian diet for bariatric cooking is that it is naturally lower in calories. Plant-based foods tend to be much lower in calories than animal-based foods, making them ideal for those looking to maintain a healthy weight. In addition, many vegetarian foods are high in fiber, which can help to keep you feeling full longer while ensuring that you get the vitamins and minerals your body needs.

A vegetarian diet can also be beneficial for those undergoing bariatric surgery because it is free of unhealthy fats, such as saturated and trans fats. These fats can be difficult to digest and can lead to digestive issues. Plant-based foods, on the other hand, are naturally low in unhealthy fats, making them easier to digest and helping to reduce the risk of digestive problems.

A vegetarian diet can also provide a wide range of health benefits. Studies have shown that people who follow a vegetarian diet tend to have lower blood pressure and cholesterol levels, as well as a lower risk of developing certain chronic diseases. Vegetarian diets are also naturally rich in vitamins and minerals, which can help to boost your overall health.

Overall, vegetarian diets can be very beneficial for bariatric cooking. They can help you to lose weight and maintain a healthy weight, while simultaneously providing you with a wide range of vitamins and minerals. Plus, they're easy to prepare and can be incredibly tasty, making them a great choice for those looking to eat healthily and enjoy their meals.

Chapter 3

10 Eating Habits After Bariatric Surgery

Eating habits after bariatric surgery are very important for successful weight loss and long-term weight maintenance. Following bariatric surgery, patients must make significant changes to their eating habits to ensure optimal health and weight loss.

It can be difficult for patients to adjust to the dietary restrictions and changes that follow bariatric surgery — but it is essential to successful outcomes. After bariatric surgery, patients must adhere to a strict diet that limits the amount of food they can consume and the types of food they can eat.

Immediately following surgery, patients are typically placed on a liquid-only diet that consists of protein shakes and sugar-free liquids. This diet helps the body recover from surgery and helps to reduce the risk of complications. After a few days, patients may move to a pureed diet that is made up of very soft, blended foods like cooked vegetables, soups, and stews.

After a few weeks, patients may be able to move to a regular diet, but it must be low in fat, sugar, and calories. Protein should be the focus of the diet, with lean sources such as skinless chicken, fish, eggs, and tofu. Fruits and vegetables should also be included in the diet.

Here are some healthy habits required to maintain a healthy lifestyle after bariatric surgery:

1. Eat slowly

Eating slowly is an important eating habit to adopt after bariatric surgery. Eating slowly gives the body more time to register fullness, reduces the risk of overeating, and helps to prevent nausea and acid reflux. Eating too quickly after bariatric surgery can cause a patient to vomit, become nauseous, or experience pain due to stretching the stomach pouch too much. Eating slowly also helps to ensure you are chewing your food thoroughly and getting the most nutrition out of the food.

Also, eating slowly helps to prevent dumping syndrome, which is a side effect of bariatric surgery where food moves too quickly through the stomach and intestines, leading to nausea, sweating, faintness, and diarrhea. Eating slowly is an important habit to practice to help ensure successful weight loss after bariatric surgery.

2. Avoid eating large meals:

Large meals can cause discomfort and can be difficult to digest after bariatric surgery. Instead, patients should focus on eating smaller, more frequent meals throughout the day.

Avoiding eating large meals after bariatric surgery is an important eating habit that can help you manage your weight and ensure successful weight loss. Eating smaller, more frequent meals allows you to better control your portion sizes and digestion, as well as reduce the risk of dumping syndrome. Dumping syndrome can occur when large amounts of food are consumed at once, resulting in nausea, vomiting, and abdominal pain. Eating smaller meals also helps to reduce hunger and can help you better meet your nutritional needs.

3. Eat protein first:

Protein is essential for healing and helping the body to recover after bariatric surgery. Patients should make sure to prioritize protein sources such as lean meats, fish, eggs, legumes, and dairy products.

Eating protein first is an important eating habit to follow after bariatric surgery. By eating protein-rich foods first, bariatric patients can ensure they are getting enough protein within their reduced calorie intake. Protein helps to increase satiety, helping patients to feel fuller for longer, and also helps to support the maintenance and growth of muscle, which is important for maintaining a healthy weight. Additionally, protein-rich foods take longer to digest, which can help to slow down the rate at which food is consumed, allowing patients to be mindful of portion sizes and avoid overeating.

4. Avoid sugar and processed foods:

Avoiding sugar and processed food as an eating habit after bariatric surgery is important for several reasons. First, sugar and processed foods can be high in calories and low in nutrition, making them poor choices for post-surgery diets.

Second, after bariatric surgery, it can be difficult for the body to digest and absorb high levels of sugar and processed foods, which can lead to nutritional deficiencies and other health problems.

Finally, consuming too much sugar and processed food can lead to weight gain, which can reverse the progress made through bariatric surgery. Eating a healthy, balanced diet full of fresh fruits and vegetables, lean proteins, and whole grains is key to maintaining a healthy weight and lifestyle after bariatric surgery.

5. Drink plenty of water:

Drinking plenty of water is an important eating habit after bariatric surgery. It helps keep the body hydrated and flush out toxins, as well as helps to reduce hunger and fill up the stomach. Water also helps to soften food in the stomach, making it easier to digest.

It also helps to prevent constipation, which is a common side effect of bariatric surgery. Finally, drinking water throughout the day encourages healthy eating habits and can help reduce cravings and overeating. You should aim to drink at least 8 glasses of water a day.

6. Avoid alcohol:

Patients should avoid drinking alcohol to ensure that their recovery is as smooth as possible.

Avoiding alcohol as an eating habit after bariatric surgery is important for some reasons. Alcohol is high in calories and can cause dehydration, which can lead to nausea and vomiting. In addition, alcohol can interfere with the absorption of nutrients, which can lead to nutrient deficiencies. Drinking alcohol can also slow down the healing process and increase the risk of complications. For these reasons, it is important to avoid alcohol after bariatric surgery.

7. Avoid drinking with meals:

Drinking too much liquid with meals can cause the stomach to stretch after bariatric surgery. Patients should wait at least 30 minutes after eating before drinking fluids.

Avoiding drinking with meals after bariatric surgery is a good eating habit to have as it can help reduce the risk of nausea and vomiting associated with drinking fluids directly after eating. Drinking fluids during or directly after a meal can also lead to a feeling of fullness that can interfere with digestion. Drinking fluids with meals can also cause the stomach pouch to stretch, which can lead to weight gain and other health issues.

8. Eat high-fiber foods:

Eating high-fiber foods can help with digestion and can help prevent constipation after bariatric surgery. Fiber helps to slow digestion, which helps to reduce the risk of dumping syndrome and keeps you feeling fuller longer. Eating high-fiber foods also helps to prevent constipation, which is common after bariatric surgery.

High-fiber foods include whole grains, fruits, vegetables, legumes, nuts, and seeds. Eating these foods in combination with lean proteins and healthy fats can help to ensure that you get the nutrition that you need after bariatric surgery.

9. Chew food thoroughly:

Chewing food thoroughly is important for helping the body to digest food properly after bariatric surgery. Patients should aim to chew each bite of food at least 30 times before swallowing.

It is especially important because patients who have had bariatric surgery have smaller stomachs, which means that food needs to be broken down into smaller pieces before it can be properly digested. Chewing food thoroughly helps break down food into smaller pieces, making it easier for the stomach to digest. Additionally, chewing food thoroughly helps to increase the amount of time it takes to eat a meal, which can help patients to slow down and eat mindfully.

10. Listen to your body:

Listening to your body as an eating habit after bariatric surgery means paying attention to hunger and satiety cues to guide your eating. After bariatric surgery, your body may require smaller meals and snacks and the ability to recognize and respond to physical cues of hunger and satiety is key.

Eating beyond fullness or ignoring hunger cues can result in vomiting or feeling uncomfortable. Eating when you are hungry and stopping when you are full is important to ensure that you are getting the nutrition your body needs while managing your weight.

Eating habits are important after bariatric surgery as they can help to ensure successful long-term weight loss results.

Chapter 4

Shopping for Vegetarian Bariatric Foods

Shopping for vegetarian bariatric foods may appear difficult at first, but if you get the hang of it, it can be a joyful and rewarding experience. There are numerous varieties of vegetarian bariatric foods available, and selecting the appropriate ones for your specific requirements might make all the difference. We'll go over some of the basics to keep in mind when shopping for vegetarian bariatric foods down below.

While looking for vegetarian bariatric foods, the first thing to consider is your nutritional needs and tastes. Depending on the sort of vegetarian bariatric diet you follow, you may need to avoid some items while emphasizing others. If you're on a vegan diet, for example, you'll need to choose items that don't contain any animal ingredients. If you adopt a lacto-ovo vegetarian diet, however, you must focus on items that include both dairy and eggs. You should also examine any food allergies or sensitivities you may have.

The nutritional composition of the foods you choose is another key element to consider while shopping for vegetarian bariatric foods. Many of these foods are specifically intended to deliver the nutrients required for weight loss and overall wellness.

Seek foods that are high in protein, low in carbs, and high in vitamins and minerals. Protein and fiber sources include whole grains and legumes such as quinoa, black beans, and lentils. Vegetables and fruits should be a staple of your diet and look for foods high in vitamins and minerals, such as dark leafy greens, carrots, and apples. Choose foods with low levels of saturated and trans fats, salt, and added sugars.

Look for calcium and vitamin D-fortified foods to guarantee the proper intake of these key elements. Finally, seek foods that are minimal in calories while yet providing the macronutrients required to maintain a healthy weight and lifestyle. This will guarantee that your vegetarian bariatric diet is as effective as possible.

While shopping for vegetarian bariatric foods, it's critical to read the labels on the products. Look for those that include thorough information on the food's nutritional content as well as any additional ingredients. This will assist you in ensuring that the food you purchase is acceptable for your diet. If you're unsure what to look for, you may always seek the advice of a nutritionist or dietitian.

While shopping for vegetarian bariatric foods, it is critical to always buy in bulk whenever possible. Purchasing a large quantity of a product in bulk is a wonderful method to save money because many retailers provide discounts for purchasing a large quantity of a product.

Bulk purchasing allows you to stock up on a large supply of vegetarian bariatric foods at once, ensuring that you have plenty for a while. This can help you save time and energy while shopping for groceries, as well as save you from running out of food.

Shopping for vegetarian bariatric meals can be difficult at first, but with a little patience and information, you'll be on your way to a healthier diet in no time. When shopping for these foods, keep the recommendations above in mind, and you'll be sure to get the appropriate cuisine for your specific needs. Eating the correct meals can make or break your weight loss attempts, so take the time to locate the ones that are appropriate for you. You can have a delicious and healthy vegetarian bariatric diet with a little effort and perseverance.

Chapter 5

Meal Planning for Vegetarian Bariatric Patients

A meal plan for a vegetarian bariatric patient should focus on high-protein plant-based sources, such as legumes, tempeh, nuts, seeds, and tofu. These foods are packed with protein and can help to fill you up without adding too many calories. It is also important to include plenty of low-calorie vegetables and fruits, such as leafy greens, broccoli, cauliflower, and berries. These can be eaten raw or cooked and can help to provide essential vitamins and minerals.

Whole grains, such as quinoa, oats, barley, and brown rice, are also important for bariatric patients, as they provide fiber, vitamins, and minerals. It is important to choose whole grains that are low in calories and high in fiber, as these can help to keep you feeling full for longer.

When cooking for a vegetarian bariatric patient, it is important to use low-calorie ingredients such as vegetable stock, low-sodium soy sauce, and herbs and spices to add flavor without adding too many calories. It is also important to avoid fried foods, added sugars, and processed foods, as these can be high in calories and low in nutrition.

It is important to include protein shakes or smoothies in your meal plan. These can provide an easy way to get in extra protein and calories without adding too many carbs. Protein powders made from plant-based sources, such as peas, hemp, and brown rice, are the best options for vegetarian bariatric patients.

By following these tips, you can create a meal plan for a vegetarian bariatric patient that is both nutritious and satisfying.

7-day Vegetarian Bariatric Meal Plan

DAY 1

Breakfast

Overnight oats with chia seeds, almond milk, and fresh or frozen berries

Ingredients:

- 1/2 cup rolled oats

- 2 tablespoons chia seeds

- 1/2 cup almond milk

- 1/4 cup fresh or frozen berries

Instructions:

1. In a bowl, mix the oats and chia seeds.

2. Pour almond milk over the mixture and stir until combined.

3. Add the berries and stir until combined.

4. Cover the bowl and refrigerate overnight.

5. In the morning, serve the oats cold or heat them in the microwave. Enjoy!

Lunch

Broccoli and cauliflower cheese soup

Ingredients:

-1 head of broccoli, cut into florets

-1 head of cauliflower, cut into florets

-1 onion, diced

-1 garlic clove, minced

-4 cups of vegetable stock

-2 teaspoons of Dijon mustard

-3/4 cup of grated cheddar cheese

-1/2 cup of cream

-Salt and pepper, to taste

Instructions:

1. In a large pot, heat a tablespoon of oil over medium heat.

2. Add the onion and garlic and cook for 5 minutes, until softened.

3. Add the broccoli and cauliflower florets, and cook for a few more minutes.

4. Add the vegetable stock and allow it to boil. Reduce the heat and simmer for 10 minutes, or until the vegetables are tender.

5. Puree the soup with an immersion blender until smooth.

6. Stir in the Dijon mustard, cheddar cheese, and cream.

7. Season to taste with salt and pepper.

8. Serve warm. Enjoy!

Snack

Celery sticks with hummus

Ingredients

- 4 celery sticks

- 1/4 cup of hummus

Instructions

1. Wash the celery sticks and dry them off with a paper towel.

2. Slice the celery sticks into 2-inch pieces.

3. Place the hummus in a small bowl and stir until it's smooth.

4. Dip the celery sticks into the hummus and enjoy!

Dinner

Baked sweet potatoes topped with black beans and avocado

Ingredients

- 2 large sweet potatoes, washed and scrubbed

- 1 tablespoon olive oil

- 1 can black beans, drained and rinsed

- 1/2 cup diced red onion

- 1 jalapeno pepper, seeded and minced (optional)

- 1/4 cup chopped cilantro

- 1/2 teaspoon cumin

- 1/2 teaspoon chili powder

- 1/2 teaspoon garlic powder

- 1/4 teaspoon salt

- 1/4 teaspoon black pepper

- 1 avocado, diced

- 2 tablespoons lime juice

Instructions

1. Preheat oven to 400°F.

2. Place sweet potatoes on a baking sheet and rub them with olive oil. Bake for 45 minutes, or until tender.

3. Meanwhile, in a large bowl, combine black beans, red onion, jalapeno (if using), cilantro, cumin, chili powder, garlic powder, salt, and black pepper. Mix until combined.

4. When sweet potatoes are done, remove from oven and top with black bean mixture.

5. In a small bowl, combine diced avocado, lime juice, and a pinch of salt.

6. Top sweet potatoes with avocado mixture and serve. Enjoy!

DAY 2

Breakfast

Scrambled eggs with bell peppers and spinach

Ingredients:

- 4 eggs

- 2 tablespoons of butter

- ½ a bell pepper (any color), diced

- ½ cup of spinach, chopped

- Salt and pepper to taste

Instructions:

1. Crack the eggs into a medium bowl and whisk until combined.

2. Melt the butter in a nonstick skillet over medium-high heat.

3. Add the bell pepper to the skillet and cook for about 2 minutes, stirring occasionally.

4. Add the spinach to the skillet and cook for another 2 minutes, stirring occasionally.

5. Pour the eggs into the skillet and stir continuously until they are scrambled and cooked through.

6. Season with salt and pepper to taste.

7. Serve the scrambled eggs with bell peppers and spinach warm.

Enjoy!

Lunch

Quinoa and black bean salad

Ingredients:

-1 cup cooked quinoa

-1 can black beans, rinsed and drained

-1/2 red onion, diced

-1 red bell pepper, diced

-1/4 cup cilantro, chopped

-2 tablespoons olive oil

-2 tablespoons lime juice

-1/2 teaspoon garlic powder

-1/2 teaspoon cumin

-Salt and pepper to taste

Instructions:

1. In a large bowl, combine the cooked quinoa, black beans, red onion, red bell pepper, and cilantro.

2. In a separate bowl, mix the olive oil, lime juice, garlic powder, cumin, and salt and pepper.

3. Pour the dressing over the quinoa and bean mixture and toss to combine.

4. Refrigerate the salad for at least 2 hours before serving to allow the flavors to meld.

5. Serve chilled or at room temperature. Enjoy!

Snack

Greek yogurt with fresh berries

Ingredients:

- 2 cups plain Greek yogurt

- 1 cup fresh berries (strawberries, blueberries, raspberries, etc.)

- 2 tablespoons honey

- 2 tablespoons toasted almonds, chopped

- 1 teaspoon vanilla extract

Instructions:

1. In a large bowl, combine the yogurt and honey. Stir until the honey is fully incorporated into the yogurt.

2. Add the fresh berries and the toasted almonds to the yogurt and honey mixture and stir to combine.

3. Add the vanilla extract and stir until combined.

4. Serve the Greek yogurt with fresh berries in individual bowls or cups. Enjoy!

Dinner

Vegetarian stir-fry with tofu, broccoli, and carrots

Ingredients:

-1 package of extra-firm tofu, drained and cubed

-1 head of broccoli, cut into florets

-2 carrots, peeled and sliced

-2 tablespoons of sesame oil

-2 cloves of garlic, minced

-2 tablespoons of soy sauce

-1 tablespoon of rice vinegar

-1 teaspoon of sugar

-Salt and pepper to taste

Instructions:

1. Heat the sesame oil in a large skillet over medium-high heat.

2. Add the tofu cubes and cook until golden brown, stirring occasionally.

3. Add the garlic, broccoli, and carrots and cook until the vegetables are tender about 5 minutes.

4. Add the soy sauce, rice vinegar, and sugar and stir to combine.

5. Season with salt and pepper to taste.

6. Serve hot. Enjoy!

DAY 3

Breakfast

Oatmeal with almond milk, banana, and walnuts

Ingredients:

- ½ cup of oats

- 1 cup of almond milk

- 1 banana, sliced

- 2 tablespoons of chopped walnuts

Instructions:

1. In a medium saucepan, bring the almond milk to a boil over medium-high heat.

2. Once boiling, add the oats and reduce the heat to low.

3. Simmer the oats for 5 minutes, stirring occasionally.

4. Remove the pan from the heat and stir in the banana slices.

5. Transfer the oatmeal to a bowl and top with chopped walnuts.

6. Serve warm and enjoy!

Lunch

Grilled vegetable wrap with hummus

Ingredients:

- 2 large whole wheat tortillas

- 1 red bell pepper, sliced

- 1 green bell pepper, sliced

- 1/2 yellow onion, sliced

- 1 small zucchini, sliced

- 1/2 cup hummus

- 2 tablespoons olive oil

- Salt and pepper to taste

Instructions:

1. Preheat a grill or grill pan to medium-high heat.

2. In a medium bowl, combine the bell peppers, onion, zucchini, and olive oil. Sprinkle with salt and pepper, then toss to combine.

3. Place the vegetables on the preheated grill and cook, stirring occasionally, until they're lightly charred and cooked through, about 5-7 minutes.

4. Meanwhile, spread each tortilla with 1/4 cup of hummus.

5. When the vegetables are cooked through, remove them from the grill and divide them between the two tortillas.

6. Wrap the tortillas into a burrito-style fold and serve. Enjoy!

Snack

Apple slices with peanut butter

Ingredients

- 2 apples

- 2 tablespoons of peanut butter

Instructions

1. Start by washing the apples.

2. Cut the apples into slim pieces.

3. Spread the peanut butter on each slice of the apple.

4. Enjoy!

Dinner

Vegetarian chili with beans, bell peppers, and tomatoes

Ingredients:

-1 tablespoon olive oil

-1 onion, chopped

-2 cloves garlic, minced

-2 bell peppers, chopped

-1 can (14.5 ounces) diced tomatoes

-1 can (15 ounces) of black beans, drained and rinsed

-1 can (15 ounces) of kidney beans, drained and rinsed

-1 can (15 ounces) corn, drained

-2 tablespoons chili powder

-1 teaspoon ground cumin

-1 teaspoon ground coriander

-1 teaspoon smoked paprika

-1 teaspoon oregano

-1 teaspoon brown sugar

-Salt and pepper, to taste

-Optional Toppings: shredded cheese, sour cream, diced avocado, chopped cilantro, lime wedges

Instructions:

1. Heat the olive oil in a large pot over medium heat.

2. Add the onion and garlic and cook until softened, about 5 minutes.

3. Add the bell peppers and cook for an additional 2 minutes.

4. Stir in the diced tomatoes, black beans, kidney beans, corn, chili powder, cumin, coriander, smoked paprika, oregano, and brown sugar.

5. Simmer for 30 minutes, stirring occasionally.

6. Season with salt and pepper to taste.

7. Serve chili with toppings of your choice. Enjoy!

DAY 4

Breakfast

Avocado toast with tomatoes and spinach

Ingredients:

- 2 slices of whole wheat bread

- 1 ripe avocado

- 1/2 cup of cherry tomatoes, halved

- 1/4 cup of spinach leaves

- 2 tsp of olive oil

- 1/4 tsp of salt

- 1/4 tsp of black pepper

- Optional: 1/4 cup of feta cheese

Instructions:

1. Toast the bread slices until lightly golden.

2. In a small bowl, mash the avocado until creamy.

3. Spread the mashed avocado over the toast slices.

4. Top the toast with the halved cherry tomatoes and spinach leaves.

5. Drizzle the olive oil over the toast and season with salt and pepper.

6. Optional: Sprinkle feta cheese over the toast.

7. Serve and enjoy!

Lunch

Lentil soup with kale

Ingredients

- 2 tablespoons olive oil

- 1 onion, diced

- 2 cloves garlic, minced

- 2 carrots, diced

- 2 celery stalks, diced

- 1 teaspoon dried thyme

- 1 teaspoon ground cumin

- 1 teaspoon smoked paprika

- 4 cups vegetable broth

- 2 cups cooked lentils

- 2 cups chopped kale

- Salt and pepper to taste

Instructions

1. Heat the olive oil in a large pot over medium heat.

2. Add the onion and garlic and cook until the onions are translucent about 5 minutes.

3. Add the carrots and celery and cook for 5 minutes more.

4. Add the thyme, cumin, and smoked paprika and cook for 1 minute.

5. Add the vegetable broth, lentils, and kale and bring to a boil.

6. Reduce the heat to low and simmer for 10 minutes.

7. Season with salt and pepper to taste.

8. Serve hot.

Snack

Roasted chickpeas

Ingredients

- 1 can chickpeas, drained and rinsed

- 2 tablespoons olive oil

- 2 teaspoons garlic powder

- 1 teaspoon smoked paprika

- 1 teaspoon ground cumin

- Salt and pepper to taste

Instructions

1. Preheat oven to 375°F.

2. Drain and rinse chickpeas and spread them on a baking sheet.

3. Drizzle with olive oil and sprinkle with garlic powder, smoked paprika, cumin, salt, and pepper.

4. Mix everything with your hands to ensure all of the chickpeas are evenly coated.

5. Bake for 30 minutes, stirring halfway through.

6. Remove from oven and let cool before serving. Enjoy!

Dinner

Zucchini noodles with pesto

Ingredients

- 3 zucchinis

- 2 cloves garlic, minced

- 1/4 cup toasted pine nuts

- 2 cups fresh basil leaves

- 1/4 cup extra-virgin olive oil

- 1/4 cup freshly grated Parmesan cheese

- Salt and freshly ground pepper, to taste

Instructions

1. Using a spiralizer, mandoline, or vegetable peeler, cut the zucchini into long, thin noodles. Set aside.

2. In a food processor or blender, combine the garlic, pine nuts, basil, olive oil, and Parmesan cheese. Pulse until a paste is formed.

3. In a large bowl, combine the zucchini noodles and pesto. Toss until the noodles are coated.

4. Season with salt and pepper, to taste.

5. Serve warm or cold. Enjoy!

DAY 5

Breakfast

Smoothie bowl with almond milk, banana, and chia seeds

Ingredients

- 2 cups almond milk

- 1 banana, peeled and sliced

- 2 tablespoons chia seeds

- 1/4 cup frozen berries (optional)

- 1/4 cup shredded coconut (optional)

Instructions

1. Place almond milk, banana, and chia seeds in a blender and blend until smooth.

2. Pour the mixture into a bowl and top with frozen berries and shredded coconut, if desired.

3. Enjoy your smoothie bowl!

Lunch

Baked sweet potato with black beans and spinach

Ingredients:

- 2 sweet potatoes

- 1 can of black beans

- 1 cup of spinach

- 2 tablespoons of olive oil

- 1 teaspoon of garlic powder

- 1 teaspoon of cumin

- Salt and pepper to taste

Instructions:

1. Preheat the oven to 400 degrees F.

2. Wash and dry the sweet potatoes, then poke a few holes in each one with a fork. Place on a baking sheet and bake for 45 minutes or until the sweet potatoes are tender.

3. While the sweet potatoes are baking, heat a skillet over medium-high heat and add the olive oil.

4. Add the black beans, spinach, garlic powder, cumin, and salt and pepper to the skillet. Cook for 5 minutes or until the spinach is wilted and the beans are warmed through.

5. Once the sweet potatoes are finished baking, slice them in half lengthwise and scoop out the flesh. Place the flesh in a bowl and mash it with a fork.

6. Divide the black bean and spinach mixture into the sweet potato halves. Top with the mashed sweet potato and bake for an additional 10 minutes.

7. Serve the baked sweet potatoes and enjoy!

Snack

Celery sticks with peanut butter

Ingredients:

-Celery sticks

-Peanut butter

Instructions:

1. Wash and cut the celery sticks into 3-4 inch pieces.

2. Spread a thin layer of peanut butter onto each celery stick.

3. Serve the celery sticks with peanut butter immediately or store them in an airtight container in the refrigerator for up to 3 days.

Enjoy!

Dinner

Vegetarian quesadillas with beans, bell peppers, and cheese

Ingredients:

- 2 tablespoons olive oil

- 1 red bell pepper, diced

- 1 green bell pepper, diced

- 1/2 onion, diced

- 1/2 teaspoon chili powder

- 1/2 teaspoon cumin

- 1/2 teaspoon garlic powder

- Salt and pepper to taste

- 1 can black beans, drained and rinsed

- 2 cups shredded cheese (cheddar or Monterey Jack)

- 8 flour tortillas

Instructions:

1. Over medium heat, in a large skillet, heat the oil.

2. Add the bell peppers, onion, chili powder, cumin, garlic powder, salt, and pepper to the skillet and cook until the vegetables are softened, about 5 minutes.

3. Add the black beans to the pan and cook for another 3-4 minutes.

4. Remove the vegetables and beans from the heat and set aside

5. Place a tortilla in the skillet and sprinkle 1/4 cup of cheese over half of the tortilla.

6. Top the cheese with one-eighth of the vegetable/bean mixture.

7. Fold the other half of the tortilla over the filling and cook until golden brown and the cheese is melted, about 3 minutes per side.

8. Remove from the heat and do the same with the ingredients left.

9. Cut the quesadillas into wedges and serve warm. Enjoy!

DAY 6

Breakfast

Omelet with mushrooms, spinach, and tomatoes

Ingredients:

- 2 eggs

- 2 tablespoons of water

- 2 tablespoons of butter

- 1 cup of sliced mushrooms

- 1/4 cup of spinach, chopped

- 1/4 cup of diced tomatoes

- Salt and pepper to taste

Instructions:

1. Beat together eggs and water in a medium bowl until combined.

2. Heat butter in a large non-stick skillet over medium-high heat.

3. Add mushrooms and sauté for a few minutes until beginning to soften.

4. Add spinach, tomatoes, and season with salt and pepper. Sauté for a few minutes more until vegetables are soft.

5. Pour egg mixture into skillet, stirring occasionally, until eggs are cooked to the desired doneness.

6. Serve an omelet with mushrooms, spinach, and tomatoes. Enjoy!

Lunch

Salad with roasted vegetables

Ingredients:

- 2 red peppers, diced

- 2 sweet potatoes, diced

- 2 zucchinis, diced

- 2 tablespoons olive oil

- 1 cup cooked quinoa

- 1 can chickpeas, drained and rinsed

- 2 cups spinach

- ½ cup crumbled feta cheese

- ¼ cup chopped fresh parsley

- 2 tablespoons balsamic vinegar

- Salt and pepper to taste

Instructions:

1. Preheat oven to 400°F.

2. Spread the diced red peppers, sweet potatoes, and zucchini on a baking sheet and drizzle with olive oil. Roast for 20-25 minutes,

stirring occasionally until vegetables are tender and lightly browned.

3. In a large bowl, combine the cooked quinoa, chickpeas, spinach, feta cheese, and parsley.

4. Add the roasted vegetables to the bowl and mix to combine.

5. Drizzle the balsamic vinegar over the top and season with salt and pepper to taste.

6. Serve the salad warm or chilled. Enjoy!

Snack

Greek yogurt with walnuts and blueberries

Ingredients:

- 2 cups plain Greek yogurt

- 1/2 cup chopped walnuts

- 1/2 cup fresh or frozen blueberries

Instructions:

1. In a medium bowl, combine the Greek yogurt and walnuts and stir until mixed.

2. Include the blueberries and stir until it mixes thoroughly.

3. Place the mixture into individual serving containers, or a single bowl if desired.

4. Serve chilled and enjoy!

Dinner

Eggplant parmesan

Ingredients:

-2 eggplants, sliced into 1/2-inch rounds

-1/2 cup all-purpose flour

-2 eggs, lightly beaten

-1 1/2 cups Italian-style bread crumbs

-1/4 cup olive oil

-2 cups marinara sauce

-1/2 cup grated Parmesan cheese

-1/2 cup shredded mozzarella cheese

Instructions:

1. Preheat oven to 375 degrees F (190 degrees C).

2. Place the flour in a shallow dish. Place the beaten eggs in a separate shallow dish. Place the bread crumbs in a third shallow dish.

3. Dip the eggplant slices into the flour, coating both sides. Dip the flour-coated eggplant slices into the beaten eggs, then dip them into the bread crumbs, coating both sides.

4. Heat the olive oil in a large skillet over medium-high heat. Add the breaded eggplant slices and cook until golden brown, about 3 minutes on each side.

5. Spread 1 cup of the marinara sauce in the bottom of a 9x13 inch baking dish. Place the cooked eggplant slices in the dish.

6. Top the eggplant slices with the remaining 1 cup of marinara sauce and sprinkle with Parmesan and mozzarella cheese.

7. Bake in the preheated oven for 25 to 30 minutes, or until the cheese is melted and bubbly.

DAY 7

Breakfast

Breakfast burrito with black beans, bell peppers, and avocado

Ingredients:

- 1/4 cup cooked black beans

- 1/4 cup diced bell peppers

- 1/4 cup diced avocado

- 2 large flour tortillas

- Shredded cheese (optional)

- Hot sauce (optional)

Instructions:

1. Heat a large skillet over medium heat.

2. Add the beans and bell peppers and cook until the bell peppers are soft, about 4 minutes.

3. Divide the bean-pepper mixture between the two tortillas.

4. Top with diced avocado and shredded cheese, if using.

5. Fold the burrito and cook in the skillet for a few minutes on each side to lightly brown the tortilla.

6. Serve with hot sauce, if desired. Enjoy!

Lunch

Spinach salad with grilled vegetables

Ingredients:

- 2 cups fresh spinach

- 1/2 cup grilled vegetables (such as peppers, zucchini, yellow squash, or eggplant)

- 2 tablespoons olive oil

- One tablespoon of balsamic vinegar

- 1 tablespoon minced fresh basil

- 1/2 teaspoon garlic powder

- Salt and pepper to taste

Instructions:

1. Preheat the grill to medium-high heat.

2. Grill the vegetables for about 5 minutes, or until tender.

3. In a large bowl, combine the spinach, grilled vegetables, olive oil, balsamic vinegar, basil, garlic powder, and salt and pepper.

4. Toss to combine.

5. Serve immediately.

Snack

Carrot sticks with hummus

Ingredients:

- 3 large carrots, cut into sticks

- 1/4 cup hummus

Instructions:

1. Heat the oven to 350°F and set a baking sheet with parchment paper.

2. Place the carrot sticks on the baking sheet and bake for 10-15 minutes, or until slightly softened.

3. Remove from the oven and let cool.

4. Serve the carrot sticks with hummus for dipping. Enjoy!

Dinner

Roasted portobello mushrooms with quinoa and steamed vegetables

Ingredients:

- 2 portobello mushrooms

- 1 cup cooked quinoa

- 1 cup steamed vegetables (such as carrots, broccoli, and/or cauliflower)

- 1 tablespoon olive oil

- Salt and pepper to taste

Instructions:

1. Heat the oven to 400 degrees Fahrenheit.

2. Clean and dry the portobello mushrooms and remove the stems. Place them on a baking sheet.

3. Drizzle the mushrooms with olive oil and season with salt and pepper.

4. Roast in the preheated oven for 20 minutes.

5. Meanwhile, cook the quinoa according to package instructions.

6. Steam the vegetables for about 5 minutes, until tender.

7. To assemble the dish, divide the quinoa between two plates and top it with the roasted mushrooms.

8. Add the steamed vegetables and enjoy!

Chapter 6

Recipes for the Pre-Surgery Diet

Breakfast

1. Veggie Omelette:

Ingredients: 2 eggs, 1/4 cup diced onion, 1/4 cup diced bell pepper, 1/4 cup diced mushrooms, 1/4 cup diced tomatoes, 1 tablespoon olive oil, salt, and pepper to taste.

Prep Time: 15 minutes

Preparation: In a medium skillet, heat the olive oil over medium heat. Add the diced onion, bell pepper, mushrooms, and tomatoes and sauté for 5 minutes until softened. In a small bowl, whisk together the eggs and season with salt and pepper. Pour the eggs into the skillet and cook for 3-4 minutes until the omelet is cooked through. Serve warm.

2. Tofu Scramble:

Ingredients: 1 block of extra firm tofu, 1/4 cup diced onion, 1/4 cup diced bell pepper, 1/4 cup diced mushrooms, 1 tablespoon olive oil, 1 teaspoon turmeric, 1 teaspoon garlic powder, salt, and pepper to taste.

Prep Time: 15 minutes

Preparation: Drain and press the block of tofu. In a medium skillet, heat the olive oil over medium heat. Add the diced onion, bell pepper, and mushrooms and sauté for 5 minutes until softened. Crumble the tofu into the skillet and season with the turmeric, garlic powder, salt, and pepper. Cook for 5-7 minutes, stirring occasionally until the tofu is cooked through. Serve warm.

3. Vegetable Frittata:

Ingredients: 4 eggs, 1/4 cup diced onion, 1/4 cup diced bell pepper, 1/4 cup diced mushrooms, 1/4 cup diced tomatoes, 1 tablespoon olive oil, salt, and pepper to taste.

Prep Time: 15 minutes

Preparation: In a medium skillet, heat the olive oil over medium heat. Add the diced onion, bell pepper, mushrooms, and tomatoes and sauté for 5 minutes until softened. In a small bowl, whisk together the eggs and season with salt and pepper. Pour the eggs into the skillet and cook for 3-4 minutes until the frittata is cooked through. Serve warm.

4. Quinoa and Veggie Bowl:

Ingredients: 1 cup cooked quinoa, 1/4 cup diced onion, 1/4 cup diced bell pepper, 1/4 cup diced mushrooms, 1/4 cup diced tomatoes, 1 tablespoon olive oil, salt, and pepper to taste.

Prep Time: 15 minutes

Preparation: In a medium skillet, heat the olive oil over medium heat. Add the diced onion, bell pepper, mushrooms, and tomatoes and sauté for 5 minutes until softened. In a medium bowl, combine the cooked quinoa and the vegetables and season with salt and pepper. Serve warm.

5. Avocado Toast:

Ingredients: 2 slices of whole wheat bread, 1/2 an avocado, 1/4 cup diced tomatoes, 1 tablespoon olive oil, salt, and pepper to taste.

Prep Time: 15 minutes

Preparation: Toast the two slices of whole wheat bread. In a small bowl, mash the avocado. Spread the mashed avocado on the toasted bread and top with the diced tomatoes. Drizzle with olive oil and season with salt and pepper. Serve warm.

6. Overnight Oats:

Ingredients: 1/2 cup oats, 1/2 cup almond milk, 1/4 cup diced apples, 1/4 cup diced peaches, 1/4 cup diced strawberries, 1 tablespoon honey, 1 tablespoon chia seeds.

Prep Time: 5 minutes

Preparation: In a medium bowl, combine the oats, almond milk, apples, peaches, strawberries, honey, and chia seeds. Stir to combine and let sit in the fridge overnight. Serve cold.

7. Smoothie Bowl:

Ingredients: 1/2 cup almond milk, 1/2 cup frozen berries, 1/4 cup diced bananas, 1 tablespoon honey, 1 tablespoon chia seeds.

Prep Time: 5 minutes

Preparation: In a blender, combine the almond milk, frozen berries, diced bananas, honey, and chia seeds. Blend until smooth. Pour into a bowl and top with additional fruit and chia seeds. Serve cold.

Lunch

1. Lentil and Kale Salad –

Ingredients: 2 cups cooked lentils, 2 cups finely chopped kale, 1/2 cup diced red onion, 1/2 cup diced green bell pepper, 1/2 cup diced cucumber, 1/4 cup olive oil, 2 tablespoons lemon juice, 1 teaspoon minced garlic, Salt and pepper to taste

Preparation: In a large bowl, combine the cooked lentils, kale, red onion, green bell pepper, and cucumber. In a small bowl, whisk together the olive oil, lemon juice, and garlic. Pour the dressing over the salad and season with salt and pepper. Toss to combine.

Preparation Time: 10 minutes

2. Roasted Vegetable Sandwich –

Ingredients: 2 slices whole wheat bread, 2 tablespoons hummus, 1/4 cup roasted vegetables (such as zucchini, eggplant, bell peppers, onions), 1/4 cup diced fresh tomatoes, 2 tablespoons crumbled feta cheese, Salt and pepper to taste

Preparation: Spread the hummus on one side of each slice of bread. Top with roasted vegetables, tomatoes, and feta cheese. Sprinkle with salt and pepper. Place the other slice of bread on top and press lightly to close.

Preparation Time: 10 minutes

3. Vegetable Quinoa Bowl –

Ingredients: 1 cup cooked quinoa, 1/2 cup diced bell peppers, 1/2 cup diced tomatoes, 1/4 cup cooked corn, 1/4 cup cooked black beans, 2 tablespoons olive oil, 2 tablespoons lime juice, 1 teaspoon minced garlic, Salt and pepper to taste

Preparation: In a large bowl, combine the cooked quinoa, bell peppers, tomatoes, corn, and black beans. In a small bowl, whisk together the olive oil, lime juice, and garlic. Pour the dressing over the bowl and season with salt and pepper. Toss to combine.

Preparation Time: 10 minutes

4. Grilled Vegetable Wrap –

Ingredients: 1 whole wheat wrap, 2 tablespoons hummus, 1/4 cup grilled vegetables (such as zucchini, eggplant, bell peppers, onions), 1/4 cup diced fresh tomatoes, 2 tablespoons crumbled feta cheese, Salt and pepper to taste

Preparation: Spread the hummus on the wrap. Top with grilled vegetables, tomatoes, and feta cheese. Sprinkle with salt and pepper. Roll up the wrap and cut it in half.

Preparation Time: 10 minutes

5. Cucumber and Avocado Salad –

Ingredients: 2 cups diced cucumber, 1/2 cup diced avocado, 1/4 cup diced red onion, 1/4 cup diced bell peppers, 2 tablespoons olive oil, 2 tablespoons lime juice, 1 teaspoon minced garlic, Salt and pepper to taste

Preparation: In a large bowl, combine the cucumber, avocado, red onion, and bell peppers. In a small bowl, whisk together the olive oil, lime juice, and garlic. Pour the dressing over the salad and season with salt and pepper. Toss to combine.

Preparation Time: 10 minutes

6. Vegetable and Bean Soup –

Ingredients: 2 cups vegetable broth, 1/2 cup diced carrots, 1/2 cup diced celery, 1/2 cup diced onion, 1/2 cup cooked white beans, 1/2 cup diced tomatoes, 1 teaspoon minced garlic, Salt and pepper to taste

Preparation: In a large saucepan, combine the vegetable broth, carrots, celery, onion, white beans, and tomatoes. Bring to a simmer over medium heat. Add the garlic and season with salt and pepper. Simmer until the vegetables are tender, about 10 minutes.

Preparation Time: 20 minutes

7. Vegetable Quiche –

Ingredients: 1 whole wheat crust, 2 cups diced vegetables (such as spinach, mushrooms, bell peppers, onions), 2 eggs, 1/2 cup milk, 1/4 cup grated cheese, 1 teaspoon minced garlic, Salt and pepper to taste

Preparation: Preheat the oven to 350 degrees F. Place the crust on a 9-inch pie plate. Spread the vegetables in the crust. In a small bowl, whisk together the eggs and milk. Pour over the vegetables and sprinkle with the cheese, garlic, salt, and pepper. Bake for 25 minutes or until the quiche is golden brown and set.

Preparation Time: 10 minutes

Dinner

1. Curried Quinoa with Roasted Sweet Potatoes:

Ingredients: 2 cups cooked quinoa, 2 small sweet potatoes, 1 tablespoon olive oil, 2 tablespoons curry powder, ½ teaspoon garlic powder, ¼ teaspoon ground turmeric, ¼ teaspoon ground cumin, ¼ teaspoon ground ginger, Salt and pepper to taste.

Preparation Method: Preheat oven to 400°F. Peel and dice sweet potatoes and place them on a baking sheet. Drizzle with oil and sprinkle with curry powder, garlic powder, turmeric, cumin, and ginger. Toss to coat and spread into a single layer. Roast for 25 minutes or until potatoes are tender. Also, cook the quinoa according to the package directions. Once cooked, add roasted sweet potatoes to the quinoa and season with salt and pepper.

Prep Time: 30 minutes.

2. Lentil Spinach Soup:

Ingredients: 1 tablespoon olive oil, 1 onion, diced, 2 cloves garlic, minced, 1 cup dry lentils, 4 cups vegetable broth, 2 cups baby spinach, 2 teaspoons dried oregano, Salt and pepper to taste.

Preparation Method: Heat oil in a large pot over medium-high heat. Add onion and garlic and cook until softened, about 5 minutes. Add lentils and stir to coat in oil. Bring to a boil after adding the vegetable broth. Reduce heat to low and simmer for 20 minutes or until lentils are tender. Stir in spinach and oregano and season with salt and pepper. Cook for an additional 5 minutes.

Prep Time: 30 minutes.

3. Eggplant and Chickpea Stew:

Ingredients: 1 tablespoon olive oil, 1 onion, diced, 2 cloves garlic, minced, 1 eggplant, diced, 1 can chickpeas, drained and rinsed, 2 cups vegetable broth, 1 can diced tomatoes, 2 teaspoons dried basil, Salt and pepper to taste.

Preparation Method: Heat oil in a large pot over medium-high heat. Add onion and garlic and cook until softened, about 5 minutes. Add eggplant and chickpeas and stir to coat in oil. Pour in vegetable broth and diced tomatoes and bring to a boil. Reduce heat to low and simmer for 20 minutes or until eggplant is tender. Basil should then be added after seasoning with salt and pepper. Cook for an additional 5 minutes.

Prep Time: 30 minutes.

4. Stuffed Portobello Mushrooms:

Ingredients: 4 large portobello mushrooms, 2 tablespoons olive oil, ½ cup cooked quinoa, ½ cup cooked brown rice, ½ cup diced tomatoes, ½ cup diced bell peppers, 2 cloves garlic, minced, 2 tablespoons fresh parsley, chopped, Salt and pepper to taste.

Preparation Method: Preheat oven to 375°F. Remove stems from mushrooms and discard. Brush mushrooms with oil and place gill side up on a baking sheet. In a medium bowl, combine quinoa, brown rice, tomatoes, bell peppers, garlic, and parsley. Season with salt and pepper. Divide the mixture between the mushrooms, pressing down to compact. Bake mushrooms for 25 minutes, or until they are soft.

Prep Time: 30 minutes.

5. Zucchini Fritters:

Ingredients: 2 zucchinis, grated, ¼ cup almond flour, 2 tablespoons chia seeds, 2 tablespoons fresh parsley, chopped, 1 teaspoon garlic powder, Salt and pepper to taste, 2 tablespoons olive oil.

Preparation Method: Place grated zucchini in a colander and sprinkle with salt. Let sit for 10 minutes, then press out excess moisture with a paper towel. In a large bowl, combine zucchini, almond flour, chia seeds, parsley, garlic powder, and salt and pepper; mix until combined. Heat oil in a large skillet over medium heat. Form the zucchini mixture into patties and add to the skillet. Cook for 4 minutes per side or until golden brown.

Prep Time: 25 minutes.

6. Greek Salad:

Ingredients: 4 cups lettuce, shredded, ½ cucumber, diced, ½ red bell pepper, diced, ½ cup Kalamata olives, ½ cup feta cheese, crumbled, 2 tablespoons olive oil, Juice of 1 lemon, 1 teaspoon dried oregano, Salt and pepper to taste.

Preparation Method: In a large bowl, combine lettuce, cucumber, bell pepper, olives, and feta. In a small bowl, whisk together olive oil, lemon juice, oregano, salt, and pepper. Pour dressing over salad and toss to combine.

Prep Time: 15 minutes.

7. Baked Tofu:

Ingredients: 1 block extra-firm tofu, ½ cup tamari or soy sauce, 2 tablespoons olive oil, 2 cloves garlic, minced, 1 teaspoon ground ginger, 1 teaspoon garlic powder, ½ teaspoon ground turmeric, Salt and pepper to taste.

Preparation Method: Preheat oven to 400°F. Slice tofu into cubes and place in a shallow baking dish. In a small bowl, whisk together tamari, olive oil, garlic, ginger, garlic powder, turmeric, salt, and pepper. Pour marinade over the tofu, tossing to coat. Bake for 25 minutes or until tofu is golden brown, flipping halfway through.

Prep Time: 30 minutes.

Chapter 7

Recipes for the Post-Surgery Diet Breakfast

1. Overnight Oats with Berries:

Ingredients: ½ cup rolled oats, ¾ cup almond milk, 1 teaspoon honey, 1 teaspoon chia seeds, ½ cup mixed berries

Preparation: In a bowl, combine the oats, milk, honey, and chia seeds. Mix until everything is combined. Place the bowl covered in the fridge overnight. In the morning, top the mixture with mixed berries.

Prep Time: 5 minutes, plus overnight soaking

2. Baked Egg Cups:

Ingredients: 4 eggs, 1 tablespoon diced red pepper, 1 tablespoon diced green pepper, 1 tablespoon diced onion, 1 teaspoon olive oil, salt, and pepper to taste

Preparation: Preheat the oven to 375 degrees Fahrenheit. Olive oil should be used to grease a muffin tray. In a mixing dish, combine the eggs, peppers, onion, olive oil, salt, and pepper. Fill each muffin cup three-quarters filled with the egg mixture. Bake for 15 minutes, or until the eggs are completely set.

Prep Time: 10 minutes

3. Banana-Almond Butter Smoothie:

Ingredients: ½ cup almond milk, ½ banana, 1 tablespoon almond butter, ½ teaspoon ground cinnamon

Preparation: In a blender, combine the almond milk, banana, almond butter, and cinnamon. Blend until smooth.

Prep Time: 5 minutes

4. Avocado Toast:

Ingredients: 1 slice whole wheat bread, ½ avocado, 1 teaspoon olive oil, 1 tablespoon diced tomatoes, salt and pepper to taste

Preparation: Toast the bread in a toaster. In a bowl, mash the avocado with a fork and spread it on the toast. Drizzle with olive oil, and top with diced tomatoes. Sprinkle with salt and pepper to taste.

Prep Time: 5 minutes

5. Egg and Quinoa Bowl:

Ingredients: ½ cup cooked quinoa, 1 egg, ½ teaspoon olive oil, 1 tablespoon diced red pepper, 1 tablespoon diced green pepper, 1 tablespoon diced onion, salt and pepper to taste

Preparation: Heat the olive oil in a skillet over medium heat. Add the peppers, onion, and salt and pepper. Cook the vegetables until soft, about 5 minutes. Add the quinoa and egg to the skillet. Cook until the egg is cooked through, about 3 minutes.

Prep Time: 10 minutes

6. Sweet Potato Pancakes:

Ingredients: 1 small sweet potato, 1 egg, ½ teaspoon baking powder, 1 tablespoon almond milk, 1 teaspoon olive oil

Preparation: In a bowl, mash the sweet potato. Add the egg, baking powder, almond milk, and olive oil. Mix until combined. Heat a skillet over medium heat, and grease with olive oil. Scoop the batter onto the skillet, forming small pancakes. Cook until golden brown, about 3 minutes per side.

Prep Time: 10 minutes

7. Veggie Frittata:

Ingredients: 2 eggs, 1 tablespoon diced red pepper, 1 tablespoon diced green pepper, 1 tablespoon diced onion, 1 tablespoon diced mushrooms, 1 teaspoon olive oil, salt, and pepper to taste

Preparation: Preheat oven to 375°F. In a skillet over medium heat, heat the olive oil. Add the peppers, onion, mushrooms, salt, and pepper to taste. Sauté for 5 minutes, or until the vegetables are softened. Whisk eggs in a mixing bowl. Pour the egg mixture into the skillet with the veggies and swirl to incorporate. Place the skillet in the oven for 10 minutes, or until the eggs are set.

Prep Time: 10 minutes

Lunch

1. Cauliflower Fried Rice:

Ingredients: 1 head of cauliflower, 1 red onion, 2 cloves of garlic, 1 red bell pepper, 3 cups of cooked brown rice, 2 tablespoons of soy sauce, 2 tablespoons of sesame oil, and 2 tablespoons of vegetable broth.

Prep Time: 10 minutes

Preparation Method: First, pulse the cauliflower in a food processor until it is in small pieces. Heat the sesame oil in a large skillet over medium heat, then add the onion and garlic and cook until they are softened. Add the bell pepper and cauliflower and cook until the vegetables are tender. Add the cooked brown rice and stir to combine. Pour in the soy sauce and broth and cook for another 5 minutes. Serve warm.

2. Mexican Quinoa Bowl:

Ingredients: 1 cup of quinoa, ¼ cup of black beans, ¼ cup of corn, 1 tomato, 1 avocado, 1 lime, 2 tablespoons of olive oil, and 1 tablespoon of chili powder.

Prep Time: 20 minutes

Preparation Method: Begin by cooking the quinoa according to package instructions. In a separate pan, heat the olive oil over medium heat, then add the black beans, corn, and chili powder. Cook the vegetables until soft. In a bowl, combine the quinoa and vegetables, then top with diced tomato and avocado slices. Squeeze the juice from the lime over the top and serve.

3. Zucchini Noodles with Tomato Sauce:

Ingredients: 2 zucchinis, 1 can of diced tomatoes, 2 cloves of garlic, 2 tablespoons of olive oil, 1 teaspoon of oregano, 1 teaspoon of basil, and 1 teaspoon of Parmesan cheese.

Prep Time: 15 minutes

Preparation Method: Begin by spiralizing the zucchini into noodles. In a separate pan, heat the olive oil over medium heat, then add the garlic and cook until it is fragrant. Add the diced tomatoes and seasonings, and cook until the sauce is thickened. Add the zucchini noodles to the sauce and cook until they are heated through. Sprinkle with Parmesan cheese and serve.

4. Roasted Veggie and Hummus Wrap:

Ingredients: 1 bell pepper, 1 zucchini, 1 red onion, 1 can of chickpeas, 1 garlic clove, ¼ cup of tahini, 2 tablespoons of olive oil, 2 tablespoons of lemon juice, and 2 whole wheat tortillas.

Prep Time: 30 minutes

Preparation Method: Preheat the oven to 425 degrees F. Chop the bell pepper, zucchini, and red onion into small pieces and spread them on a baking sheet. Drizzle with olive oil and season with salt and pepper. Roast in the oven for 20-25 minutes until vegetables are tender. Meanwhile, make the hummus by blending the chickpeas, garlic, tahini, olive oil, and lemon juice in a food processor. To assemble the wraps, spread the hummus onto the tortillas and top them with the roasted vegetables. Fold the tortillas and enjoy.

5. Eggplant Parmesan:

Ingredients: 1 eggplant, 1 cup of breadcrumbs, 1 teaspoon of Italian seasoning, ½ cup of grated Parmesan cheese, ¼ cup of olive oil, and 1 jar of marinara sauce.

Prep Time: 40 minutes

Preparation Method: Preheat the oven to 350 degrees F. Cut the eggplant into ½-inch thick pieces. In a shallow bowl, combine the breadcrumbs, Italian seasoning, and Parmesan cheese. Dip the eggplant slices in the breadcrumb mixture to coat on both sides. Heat the olive oil in a large skillet over medium heat, then add the eggplant slices and cook until they are golden brown on both sides. Place the eggplant slices on a baking sheet and top with the marinara sauce. Sprinkle with more Parmesan cheese and bake in the oven for 20 minutes. Serve warm.

6. Stuffed Sweet Potatoes:

Ingredients: 2 sweet potatoes, 1 can of black beans, 1 cup of cooked quinoa, 1 teaspoon of chili powder, 1 teaspoon of cumin, 1 tablespoon of olive oil, 1 avocado, and 1 lime.

Prep Time: 45 minutes

Preparation Method: Preheat the oven to 400 degrees F. Pierce the sweet potatoes with a fork and bake in the oven for 40 minutes. Meanwhile, heat the olive oil in a large skillet over medium heat, then add the black beans, quinoa, chili powder, and cumin. Cook until everything is well heated. When the potatoes are done, cut them in half and scoop out the insides. Place the potato flesh in the skillet with the beans and quinoa, then mash together and stir to combine. Stuff the potatoes with the mixture and top with diced avocado and a squeeze of lime juice. Serve warm.

7. Baked Cauliflower Nuggets:

Ingredients: 1 head of cauliflower, 1 cup of panko breadcrumbs, ¼ cup of grated Parmesan cheese, 1 teaspoon of garlic powder, 1 teaspoon of Italian seasoning, and 2 tablespoons of olive oil.

Prep Time: 25 minutes

Preparation Method: Preheat the oven to 400 degrees F. Make tiny florets out of the cauliflower. In a shallow bowl, combine the panko breadcrumbs, Parmesan cheese, garlic powder, and Italian seasoning. Dip the cauliflower florets in the breadcrumb mixture to coat on all sides. Place the cauliflower on a baking sheet and drizzle with olive oil. Bake in the oven for 20 minutes until golden brown. Enjoy!

Dinner

1. Vegetable Stir-Fry with Quinoa:

Ingredients: 2 cups cooked quinoa, 1 red bell pepper, 1 yellow bell pepper, 2 cups broccoli florets, 2 tablespoons olive oil, 2 cloves garlic, 2 tablespoons low-sodium soy sauce, 2 tablespoons rice vinegar, Sesame seeds (optional).

Prep Time: 10 minutes

Preparation Method: Heat olive oil in a large skillet over medium heat. Add garlic and stir-fry until fragrant. Add bell peppers and broccoli and stir-fry for 3-4 minutes. Add quinoa and stir-fry for an additional 2-3 minutes. Stir in the soy sauce and rice vinegar to mix. Cook for another 1-2 minutes. Serve heated with sesame seeds on top (optional).

2. Baked Zucchini and Eggplant Parmesan:

Ingredients: 2 zucchini, 2 eggplants, 1 jar of low-sodium marinara sauce, ¼ cup low-fat Parmesan cheese, 2 tablespoons olive oil, 2 cloves garlic, 1 teaspoon oregano, 1 teaspoon basil, Salt and pepper to taste.

Prep Time: 20 minutes

Preparation Method: Preheat oven to 375 degrees Fahrenheit. Slice zucchini and eggplant into ½ inch slices and lay on a baking sheet. Drizzle with olive oil and season with salt, pepper, oregano, and basil. Bake for 15 minutes. Heat marinara sauce in a pan over medium heat. Include garlic and cook for extra 2 minutes. Remove vegetables from the oven and layer them in an oven-safe dish. Top with marinara sauce and sprinkle with Parmesan cheese. Bake for 15 minutes more.

3. Lentil and Spinach Soup:

Ingredients: 1 cup lentils, 4 cups low-sodium vegetable broth, 2 cups spinach, 2 cloves garlic, 2 tablespoons olive oil, 2 tablespoons lemon juice, ½ teaspoon cumin, Salt and pepper to taste.

Prep Time: 10 minutes

Preparation Method: Heat olive oil in a large pot over medium heat. Add garlic and sauté for 2 minutes. Add lentils and broth and bring to a boil. Reduce heat to low and simmer for 20 minutes. Add spinach, lemon juice, cumin, salt, and pepper. Simmer for an additional 10 minutes. Serve warm.

4. Sweet Potato and Kale Salad:

Ingredients: 2 large sweet potatoes, 2 cups kale, 2 tablespoons olive oil, 2 tablespoons balsamic vinegar, 2 cloves garlic, 1 teaspoon honey, Salt and pepper to taste.

Prep Time: 10 minutes

Preparation Method: Preheat oven to 375 degrees Fahrenheit. Peel and cube sweet potatoes and lay them on a baking sheet. Drizzle with olive oil and bake for 30 minutes. In a skillet over medium heat, heat the olive oil. Add garlic and sauté for 2 minutes. Add kale and cook for an additional 2 minutes. Remove sweet potatoes from the oven and add to the pan. Add balsamic vinegar, honey, salt, and pepper, and cook for an additional 2 minutes. Serve warm.

5. Black Bean and Quinoa Burrito Bowl:

Ingredients: 1 can black beans, 2 cups cooked quinoa, 1 red bell pepper, 1 yellow bell pepper, 2 tablespoons olive oil, 2 cloves garlic, 2 tablespoons low-sodium taco seasoning, 1 avocado, 1 lime, Salt and pepper to taste.

Prep Time: 10 minutes

Preparation Method: Heat olive oil in a large skillet over medium heat. Add garlic and stir-fry until fragrant. Add bell peppers and black beans and stir-fry for 3-4 minutes. Add quinoa and taco seasoning and stir to combine. Cook for an additional 1-2 minutes. Serve in individual bowls and top with diced avocado and a squeeze of lime.

6. Roasted Vegetable Quinoa Bowl:

Ingredients: 2 cups cooked quinoa, 1 red bell pepper, 1 yellow bell pepper, 2 cups broccoli florets, 2 tablespoons olive oil, 2 cloves garlic, 2 tablespoons low-sodium soy sauce, 2 tablespoons balsamic vinegar, Salt and pepper to taste.

Prep Time: 10 minutes

Preparation Method: Preheat oven to 375 degrees Fahrenheit. Slice bell peppers and lay them on a baking sheet. Season with salt and pepper and drizzle with olive oil. 15 minutes in the oven. In a large skillet over medium heat, heat the olive oil. Stir in the garlic until fragrant. Stir-fry the broccoli for 3-4 minutes. Stir in the quinoa and cook for another 2-3 minutes. Stir in the soy sauce and balsamic vinegar to mix. Cook for another 1-2 minutes. Serve hot.

7. Baked Tofu with Roasted Vegetables:

Ingredients: 2 cups cubed firm tofu, 1 red bell pepper, 1 yellow bell pepper, 2 cups broccoli florets, 2 tablespoons olive oil, 2 cloves garlic, 2 tablespoons low-sodium soy sauce, 2 tablespoons balsamic vinegar, Salt and pepper to taste.

Prep Time: 10 minutes

Preparation Method: Preheat oven to 375 degrees Fahrenheit. Place cubed tofu on a baking sheet and bake for 15 minutes. Heat olive oil in a large skillet over medium heat. Add garlic and stir-fry until fragrant. Add bell peppers and broccoli and stir-fry for 3-4 minutes. Add soy sauce and balsamic vinegar and stir to combine. Cook for an additional 1-2 minutes. Serve tofu with roasted vegetables and season with salt and pepper to taste.

Chapter 8

Mouth-watering Snack Recipes

1. Avocado Toast:

Ingredients: 2 slices of whole wheat bread, ½ avocado, 1 teaspoon of lemon juice, 1 teaspoon of olive oil, salt, and pepper to taste.

Preparation: Toast the bread and spread the mashed avocado over it. Drizzle with olive oil and lemon juice, and season with salt and pepper.

Prep Time: 5 minutes

2. Zucchini Chips:

Ingredients: 2 zucchinis, 2 tablespoons of olive oil, salt, and pepper to taste.

Preparation: Heat oven to 375 degrees Fahrenheit. Slice the zucchini into ¼-inch thick slices. Place the slices on a baking sheet lined with parchment paper and brush with olive oil. Sprinkle with salt and pepper and bake for 25-30 minutes or until golden brown and crispy.

Prep Time: 15 minutes

3. Cucumber Salad:

Ingredients: 2 cucumbers, 1 tablespoon of olive oil, 1 tablespoon of lemon juice, salt, and pepper to taste.

Preparation: Slice the cucumbers into thin slices and place them in a bowl. Drizzle with olive oil and lemon juice and season with salt and pepper.

Prep Time: 10 minutes

4. Baked Sweet Potato Fries:

Ingredients: 2 sweet potatoes, 2 tablespoons of olive oil, salt, and pepper to taste.

Preparation: Heat oven to 400 degrees Fahrenheit. Slice the sweet potatoes into ½-inch thick slices. Place the slices on a baking sheet lined with parchment paper and brush with olive oil. Sprinkle with salt and pepper and bake for 20-25 minutes or until golden brown and crispy.

Prep Time: 20 minutes

5. Roasted Cauliflower:

Ingredients: 1 head of cauliflower, 2 tablespoons of olive oil, salt, and pepper to taste.

Preparation: Preheat oven to 400 degrees F. Cut the cauliflower into bite-sized florets and place it on a baking sheet lined with parchment paper. Season with salt and pepper and drizzle with olive oil. 25-30 minutes, or until golden brown.

Prep Time: 10 minutes

6. Hummus and Veggies:

Ingredients: ¼ cup of hummus, 2 carrots, 1 bell pepper, 1 cucumber.

Preparation: Slice the carrots, bell pepper, and cucumber into thin slices. Serve with hummus for dipping.

Prep Time: 10 minutes

7. Fruit Salad:

Ingredients: 1 apple, 1 banana, 1 orange, 1 cup of blueberries.

Preparation: Peel and dice the apple, banana, and orange. Place in a bowl with the blueberries and gently stir to combine.

Prep Time: 5 minutes

Captivating Dessert Recipes

1. Chocolate Chip Protein Mug Cake:

Ingredients: ¼ cup all-purpose flour, 2 tablespoons sugar-free chocolate chips, 2 tablespoons low-fat plain yogurt, 1 tablespoon protein powder, 2 tablespoons almond milk, ½ teaspoon baking powder, Pinch of salt

Preparation: In a bowl, mix the flour, protein powder, baking powder, and salt. Add in the yogurt, almond milk, and chocolate chips and stir until a thick batter forms. Grease a mug with cooking spray and pour the batter into it. Microwave the mug cake for 1 minute and 30 seconds. Allow the mug cake to cool before serving.

Prep Time: 2 minutes

2. Sugar-Free Banana Bread:

Ingredients: 1 large banana, 1/2 cup almond flour, 1/4 cup sugar-free sweetener, 1/4 teaspoon baking soda, 1/4 teaspoon baking powder, 1/4 teaspoon ground cinnamon, 2 large eggs, 2 tablespoons olive oil

Preparation: Preheat oven to 350° F. Mash the banana in a large bowl. Add the almond flour, sweetener, baking soda, baking powder, and cinnamon and stir together. Add the eggs and olive oil and stir until combined. Grease a loaf pan with cooking spray and pour the batter into it. Bake for 25-30 minutes, or until a toothpick inserted into the center comes out clean. Allow the banana bread to cool before serving.

Prep Time: 10 minutes

3. Apple Crisp:

Ingredients: 4 cups thinly sliced apples, 1/4 cup sugar-free sweetener, 1/2 teaspoon ground cinnamon, 2 tablespoons rolled oats, 2 tablespoons almond flour, 2 tablespoons softened butter

Preparation: Preheat oven to 375° F. Grease an 8-inch baking dish with cooking spray and add the sliced apples. In a small bowl, mix the sweetener, cinnamon, oats, and almond flour. Sprinkle the mixture evenly over the apples. Dot the top with the butter. Bake for 20-25 minutes, or until the top is golden brown and the apples are tender. Allow the apple crisp to cool before serving.

Prep Time: 10 minutes

4. Protein Blondie Bites:
Ingredients: 1/4 cup almond butter, 1/4 cup pumpkin puree, 2 tablespoons sugar-free sweetener, 1/4 cup protein powder, 1 teaspoon vanilla extract, 1/4 teaspoon baking soda

Preparation: Preheat oven to 350° F. In a bowl, mix the almond butter, pumpkin puree, sweetener, protein powder, vanilla extract, and baking soda. Grease a mini muffin tin with cooking spray and spoon the batter into the cups. Bake for 10-12 minutes, or until the blondie bites are golden brown and a toothpick inserted into the center comes out clean. Allow the blondie bites to cool before serving.

Prep Time: 10 minutes

5. Coconut Macaroons:

Ingredients: 1/2 cup shredded coconut, 2 tablespoons sugar-free sweetener, 1/2 teaspoon vanilla extract, 1 large egg white

Preparation: Preheat oven to 350° F. In a bowl, mix the shredded coconut, sweetener, and vanilla extract. Whisk the egg white until frothy and fold it into the coconut mixture. Grease a baking sheet with cooking spray and drop the coconut mixture by the tablespoon onto the sheet. Bake for 12-15 minutes, or until golden brown. Allow the coconut macaroons to cool before serving.

Prep Time: 10 minutes

6. Protein Pancakes:

Ingredients: 1/2 cup all-purpose flour, 1 scoop protein powder, 1 teaspoon baking powder, 1/4 teaspoon ground cinnamon, 1/4 teaspoon ground nutmeg, 1/4 cup low-fat plain yogurt, 2 tablespoons almond milk, 1 large egg

Preparation: In a bowl, mix the flour, protein powder, baking powder, cinnamon, and nutmeg. In a separate bowl, whisk together the yogurt, almond milk, and egg. Slowly add the wet ingredients to the dry ingredients and stir until a thick batter forms. Grease a skillet with cooking spray and drop the batter by the tablespoon onto the skillet. Cook the pancakes for 1-2 minutes on each side, or until golden brown. Serve the pancakes with your favorite toppings.

Prep Time: 10 minutes

7. Avocado Fudge Brownies:

Ingredients: 1 large ripe avocado, 1/4 cup sugar-free sweetener, 1/4 cup cocoa powder, 1 teaspoon vanilla extract, 1/4 cup protein powder, 2 tablespoons melted butter

Preparation: Preheat oven to 350° F. In a food processor, add the avocado, sweetener, cocoa powder, vanilla extract, and protein powder and blend until smooth. Add the melted butter and blend until combined. Grease an 8-inch baking dish with cooking spray and pour the batter into it. Bake for 15-20 minutes, or until a toothpick inserted into the center comes out clean. Allow the brownies to cool before serving.

Prep Time: 10 minutes

Refreshing Smoothies

1. Pineapple Peach Smoothie – Prep Time: 5 minutes

Ingredients: 1 cup frozen pineapple, ½ cup frozen peaches, ½ cup orange juice, ¼ cup low-fat Greek yogurt, ½ banana, ½ teaspoon honey

Preparation: Place all ingredients in a blender and blend until smooth.

2. Carrot Cake Smoothie – Prep Time: 5 minutes

Ingredients: ½ cup carrot juice, ½ cup plain low-fat yogurt, ½ banana, ¼ cup rolled oats, 2 tablespoons honey, ¼ teaspoon ground cinnamon

Preparation: Place all ingredients in a blender and blend until smooth.

3. Mango Coconut Smoothie – Prep Time: 5 minutes

Ingredients: 1 cup frozen mango chunks, ¼ cup coconut milk, ¼ cup plain low-fat yogurt, 2 tablespoons honey

Preparation: Place all ingredients in a blender and blend until smooth.

4. Strawberry Banana Smoothie – Prep Time: 5 minutes

Ingredients: 1 cup frozen strawberries, ½ banana, ½ cup plain low-fat yogurt, ½ cup almond milk, 2 tablespoons honey

Preparation: Place all ingredients in a blender and blend until smooth.

5. Blueberry Almond Smoothie – Prep Time: 5 minutes

Ingredients: 1 cup frozen blueberries, ½ cup almond milk, ¼ cup plain low-fat yogurt, 1 tablespoon almond butter, 2 tablespoons honey

Preparation: Place all ingredients in a blender and blend until smooth.

6. Apple Pie Smoothie – Prep Time: 5 minutes

Ingredients: 1 cup diced apple, ½ cup apple juice, ¼ cup plain low-fat yogurt, 1 teaspoon honey, ¼ teaspoon ground cinnamon

Preparation: Place all ingredients in a blender and blend until smooth.

7. Chocolate Avocado Smoothie – Prep Time: 5 minutes

Ingredients: ½ avocado, ½ banana, ½ cup almond milk, 2 tablespoons cocoa powder, 2 tablespoons honey

Preparation: Place all ingredients in a blender and blend until smooth.

Chapter 9

Supplementation

Vegetarian bariatric cooking can be a challenge for those who are trying to lose weight, as it can be difficult to get enough of the essential vitamins and minerals needed for a healthy diet. Supplementation is an important part of vegetarian bariatric cooking, as it helps to ensure that all of the essential nutrients are being provided.

When it comes to vegetarian bariatric cooking, the most important nutrient to supplement is protein. Protein is a key component in helping to build and maintain muscle, and it also helps to keep you feeling full. Plant-based proteins such as soy, quinoa, and lentils are good sources of protein, but they may not provide all of the essential amino acids that are needed for optimal health. Supplements such as whey protein, hemp protein, and pea protein can help to provide the complete range of essential amino acids.

It is also important to supplement with omega-3 fatty acids for vegetarian bariatric cooking. Omega-3 fatty acids are essential fatty acids that are needed for optimal health, but they are not found in plant-based sources. Supplements such as flaxseed oil and fish oil can provide the necessary omega-3s, and they can also help to reduce inflammation and improve heart health.

In addition to protein and omega-3s, it is also important to supplement with vitamins and minerals. Vegetarian bariatric cooking can be low in some essential vitamins and minerals, such as iron, calcium, and vitamin B12. Iron is important for red blood cell formation, calcium is important for bone health, and vitamin B12 is important for energy production. Supplements such as iron tablets, calcium tablets, and B12 tablets can help to ensure that you are getting enough of these essential vitamins and minerals.

Finally, it is important to supplement with fiber for vegetarian bariatric cooking. Fiber helps to keep you feeling full and can help to reduce cholesterol levels. Fiber can be found in many plant-based sources, such as oats, beans, and fruits, but supplements such as psyllium husk powder and chia seeds can help to ensure that you are getting enough fiber in your diet.

Supplementation is an important part of vegetarian bariatric cooking, as it helps to ensure that all of the essential vitamins and minerals are being provided. Supplements such as protein powders, omega-3 fatty acids, vitamins and minerals, and fiber can help to ensure that you are getting the nutrition you need for optimal health and weight loss.

Meal Replacement

Meal replacement is an important part of bariatric cooking, especially for vegetarians. It can provide a convenient and nutritious way to meet your daily nutritional needs. Meal replacements can help you get the necessary protein, vitamins, and minerals you need to maintain healthy weight loss.

Meal replacements are typically high-protein, low-calorie shakes, bars, or other products that can be used as a substitute for a meal. They are often fortified with vitamins and minerals and typically contain between 200 and 300 calories. Meal replacements can also come in the form of meal replacement bars, soups, and entrees.

Vegetarian meal replacements are especially important for bariatric cooking, as they provide an easy way to get the necessary nutrients without having to worry about the animal products found in traditional meals. Vegetarian meal replacements often contain plant-based proteins, such as soy, lentils, and quinoa, along with other nutritious ingredients, such as nuts, seeds, fruits, and vegetables. They are also often fortified with vitamins and minerals and can help meet the dietary needs of vegetarians who may not be able to get the necessary nutrients from their diets.

When choosing a meal replacement, it is important to look for one that is fortified with vitamins and minerals and is high in protein, and low in calories. It is also important to read the nutrition label to make sure that the meal replacement meets your dietary needs. If you are a vegetarian, it is important to look for meal replacements that are specifically made for vegetarians.

Meal replacements can be a great addition to a bariatric cooking plan. They provide a convenient and nutritious way to meet your daily nutritional needs while providing the necessary protein and vitamins and minerals that are often lacking in traditional vegetarian diets. With careful consideration, meal replacements can be an important part of a healthy bariatric cooking plan.

Conclusion

The vegetarian bariatric diet is a great way to lose weight and maintain a healthy lifestyle. By cutting out animal products and replacing them with nutritious plant-based foods, you can reduce your overall calorie intake and improve your health. Not only will you be able to shed pounds, but you'll also benefit from the long-term health benefits that come with eating a vegetarian diet. With the right combination of vegetables, fruits, legumes, whole grains, nuts, and seeds, you can create a balanced diet that provides all the necessary nutrients your body needs.

Making the switch to a vegetarian bariatric diet can be a challenge, but with a little commitment and determination, you can make it work. Start by slowly reducing animal products in your diet and adding more plant-based foods. Be sure to include plenty of fiber-rich foods such as beans, lentils, and whole grains, as well as healthy fats like nuts and seeds. Aim for variety in your diet and strive to make every meal colorful and flavorful.

By following a vegetarian bariatric diet, you can not only lose weight, but you can also improve your overall health and well-being.

You'll be able to enjoy delicious and satisfying meals that are both nutritious and satisfying. With a little bit of effort and dedication, you can create a lasting lifestyle change and enjoy the benefits of a healthy, vegetarian diet.

Cheers to a healthier and greener lifestyle !!

Printed in Great Britain
by Amazon